# How to Lose Thigh Fat

# Everything You Need to Know to Have a Slim and Sexy Leg

Kristy John

# Copyright

# Terms of Use

Any information provided in this book is through the author's interpretation. The author has done strenuous work to reassure the accuracy of this subject. If you wish you attempt any of the practices provided in this book, you are doing so with your own responsibility. The author will not be held accountable for any misinterpretations or misrepresentations of the information provided here.

All information provided is done so with every effort to represent the subject, but does not guarantee that your life will change. The author shall not be held liable for any direct or indirect damages that result from reading this book.

# Contents

# Introduction

Having thin long legs is a must for most women.

In fact, it's probably in their top five must have for body structure. Of course, who can blame them? Even men are attracted to women with thin thighs and long legs.

Unfortunately, not all women are born with the long legs that they desire. There are some women who are as short as five feet and as tall as six feet.

However, even when height cannot be altered, thinness can. So, for all the ladies out there that is searching for a solution to get rid of your thigh fat, this is it.

Before starting, you should familiarize yourself with a few facts.

If this is the first time you've started a diet then this is good to keep in mind.

The two key terms that you want to always keep in mind when you engage in any diet is fat and muscle because no matter what type of diet you chose it will always include the terms fat and muscle.

When you want to lose weight you want to get rid of the fat inside your body. So, in order to get rid of fat, you need muscles and in order to gain muscles, you need to exercise.

It's a simple straightforward solution. However, if you were to take a break from exercising, your muscles will once again turn back to fat.

Thus, your efforts will be wasted. That is why you have to be consistent with the diet program, which is why you can't stop once you start.

It's a lifetime program that will not only give you the results you want but also improves your health. In the end, you're killing two birds with one stone.

# Chapter 1 - The Big Step

The hardest step to take when you want to start anything in life is the first step.

Why?

Because that's when procrastination starts to kick in the hardest.

The longer you wait to start what you plan to start, the harder it will be for you to actually start it.

Eventually, you're going to end up locking that idea of yours into a box and leaving it alone and untouched until, for some miraculous reason, you want to restart what you've never started.

Fortunately, for this type of program, you can't do that. Well you technically can, but why give up before you've taken the first step?

Think about it. What was your goal before you started reading this book?

Now what is your goal now? The same, correct?

You were already motivated enough to start learning so why not continue to motivate yourself by taking the next step?

When you make a goal for yourself it's going to be hard to reach that goal, especially if it's a long term goal.

Each step you take towards that goal brings you closer to it. Don't start to think that it's another step that you have to take to get what you want.

Think of it as a step that brings you closer to achieve what you've started. The most important aspect of being able to achieve any goal is to be positive and continue to strive for the better.

If you want to be able to achieve the thin thighs that you've always wanted then you have to stay motivated and on track.

Don't continue in one direction if you've made a wrong turn. In your road, U-turns are not illegal. Also, don't think that it's smooth sailing when you've jumped on the boat.

You're bound to run into one or two icebergs here and there throughout the program, but that's how dieting works.

That's how you improve for the better. Plateaus aren't there because it wants to get in your way. It's there because it wants you to succeed as a better person.

Since this is a life long program, you want to be able to maintain it for as long as you live. Now, it's common to want to put less effort into what you're doing once you've achieved the results that you want.

Unfortunately, all good things must come to an end without proper care. That means that if you slack off then all your previous efforts will be wasted.

You have to remember that even after you've achieved your goal your new goal should be to maintain it.

Always stay motivated no matter what happens. Remember, the same amount of work you do to obtain the thin thighs that you want will require the same amount of work that you'll have to do to maintain those thin thighs. It's not going to be easy but it's going to be worth it.

A good aspect to keep in mind during the program is the fact that you should have fun. Procrastination appears when you are unmotivated to do something that you find boring.

Therefore, in order to find motivation and to stop yourself from procrastinating, you should try to make the program more into a fun activity rather than something that you feel compelled to doing order to get what you want.

If your goal is already hard to reach, why not try to have fun in the process. There is no harm in it and it makes the program twice as easy and less painful for you to do.

You have to remember that when you start exercising you will have to be outside where people are.

If you're the type that wants company when you leave the house then its best if you try to look for a friend who is willing to exercise with you.

The buddy system is a fun way to get you to exercise, especially when you have a friend that will help keep you entertained.

Be careful when choosing a friend that enjoys embarrassing you in public. If you're the shy type then I suggest you prepare yourself.

If anything, go along with their jokes. You might be in public but as long as you're having fun that's all that matters.

There are also plenty of other ways to stay motivated in the program. It's just whatever fits you the most.

You want to be able to feel comfortable throughout the program but you also want to be able to leave your comfort zone and experience new things that you haven't before.

Most importantly, you have to remember that it's a dedicated working process, which means that you have to plan ahead of schedule and work hard in order to accomplish what you want to accomplish.

By taking the first, and big, step into the program you have to concentrate and focus on what you're doing.

Willpower will not bring you very far in to the program. If anything, you'll last for a few months and you're done.

You have to work even when you don't feel like it. It doesn't mean that you have to give 100% effort every single day, but do try to give more than 80%.

**Making Goals:**

Making goals are as important as changing yourself. Goals usually come first before the change because in order to reach your goals, you would have to make some sort of change to yourself.

It doesn't mean that you have to constantly change for every goal you make, but there is always an aspect about yourself that can always improve for the better.

When you start establishing your goals, think about what you want out of it. Think about how it can benefit you and why you would want to accomplish that goal.

It's highly recommended to ignore the setbacks of that goal. When there's a pro, there's always a con.

Chances are, your idea is going to have a negative aspect about it that you don't like.

Most likely, if you are going to focus on that negative aspect rather than the positive aspect then you won't make it very far with your goal.

This is why positivity is especially important in life. Negativity is the biggest obstacle in life and it can stop you from achieving your goals completely if you allow it to.

A good goal is a detailed goal. When you first decide what it is that you want to accomplish, you need to plan it out.

That doesn't mean you have to pull out a fancy calendar and start planning every single detail of your daily life.

Just be specific with what you want. Ask yourself some basic questions like how you will be able to achieve your goal and what would you have to do in order to accomplish that goal.

Once you're done, answer them. You can be as specific as you want with your planning as long as you've answered the necessary questions needed to achieve your goal.

Simply stating that you want to do something isn't going to cut it if you don't know where to start. Plan your route and make your way to point B.

**Changing Yourself:**

Change is inevitable and sometimes it is necessary. That doesn't mean that change is going to happen overnight.

Changing requires time and effort. You cannot simply change if you do not want to change and, at the same time, you cannot force yourself to change.

The reason why change is such a long and tedious process is because you need time to adapt to those changes.

If any changes were to happen too quickly in your life then you would feel overwhelmed by it all and it will be more difficult for you to cope with it both mentally and physically.

Often times, changes can also be considered as a habit.

The reason why is because your body or your mind has become accustomed to whatever you have been doing.

That means that bad changes can lead to bad habits and good chances can lead to good habits.

Now you might think that habits may not be much of a big deal but it can be, especially if it takes up a big portion of your life.

This program would be an example of a life long habit. You want to make this program into a habit.

It will not only give you the results you want but you will also be a much healthier person than what you were before.

Note that it might take about one month to break into your new habit. As the saying goes, "Old habits die hard." So you need to kill off your old habits before you can bring in a new one.

Also, get into the habit of constantly encouraging yourself because it will help you a lot, especially if you were a pessimistic person from the beginning.

Negative thinking can only lead to more negative thinking. You want to rid yourself of this poor habit before you start the program because if that negativity continues then you will have a very hard time keeping up with the program.

In addition to that, you may even give up in the long run because your motivation might start to die out.

You have to constantly keep yourself in check on a daily basis.

You have to take note of how you feel and how you react to certain situations. Often times, you may know what you are doing and you may realize that what you're doing isn't what you should be doing, but you do it anyways because you can't deny yourself.

The point of being aware of your actions is the fact that you can change those actions when you need to and not when you feel like it.

**Focusing on Your Goal:**

So you want thinner thighs? You have to work for it.

As of now, your goal is to achieve the thin thighs that you want. This is the part where you start to shape yourself up.

Start thinking positive and start boosting up your motivation. It's important to control to your thoughts.

You want to be honest with yourself but you also want to stay clear from any negative traits that you may pick up along the process.

Your thoughts can reflect your whole success if you let it. You are bound to make mistakes during the program and it is normal to do so.

In fact, mistakes are good to make during the early stages of the program because you are still able to learn and fix those mistakes before they can get out of hand later on.

Remember, any mistakes that you've made in the past can be fixed in the future. That means that any mistakes that you've made yesterday and be fixed today.

When you're engaging yourself into the thin thighs program you are basically engaging yourself in a type of dieting program.

If you've never went through a diet program and this is your first them then it's important for you to know that you have to step out of your comfort zone.

That doesn't necessarily mean that you have to feel uncomfortable throughout the whole program.

Dieting is a slow process, which means that you will have to slowly move away from your comfort zone.

Take baby steps each day. Even if you want to rush it doesn't mean that your body wants to.

In order to maintain a healthy lifestyle and getting the thin thighs that you want, you need to take it slowly.

If you work too quickly then you will not only be overwhelmed, but you will also have a higher chance of inflicting damages to your body.

Remember, a fast diet is an unhealthy diet.

Try to rid yourself of any possible distractions that can stray you away from your goal.

This means no fast foods at all. Try to limit the amount of times you eat out, if you do in the first place.

Try to limit the amount of food that you eat during social gatherings because, chances are, there is going to be a lot of unhealthy junk food that is going to be laid out for you.

The list can go on but these are the few that you should keep in mind. The point is that you should stay clear from unhealthy foods period.

The sooner you start to adapt yourself to eating healthy foods the easier it will be for you resist unhealthy foods.

Be wary of your mood. You may not realize it but your mood can play a big impact on your actions.

If you're the type that eats out of stress, boredom, or convenience then it's about time you stop that habit of yours.

Usually, when you start to have cravings, you're going to end up eating something unhealthy.

It's rare for anyone to crave healthy food, which is why dieting is such a complicated process for some people.

Be careful of being tempted also. It can be risky to tell some of your friends or family that you are planning on dieting because they can really go out of their way to tempt you to eat what you are trying to stay away from.

The best method is to ignore them and, in the case where they start to rub those unhealthy foods in front of your face, it's about time to reevaluate your relationship with them.

**Keeping Track:**

In order to succeed in achieving your goals throughout the thin thighs program, you need to keep a journal of your progress.

Now that may sound a little hard to do and it may sound like a lot of work, but it will be worth it.

Keeping a journal can be a lot of work, but only when you believe that it will be.

The only hard work that you have to do when keeping a journal is the fact that you have to write in it constantly.

You have to keep your life updated in a small, compact, already organized book. There will be times when you will feel lazy enough that you won't want to record anything for the day.

That is a common feeling, but that doesn't mean that you should follow your emotions. Even when you know that you have a good memory, you should record your progress immediately.

You don't know what's going to happen in the future and you don't know if you might forget which is why it's best to do it now than to do it later.

If you think about it, it really isn't difficult to do. Recording your daily progress takes less than three minutes to do unless if you find the will to procrastinate and extend those short three minutes.

You can even record your progress while you are eating, or before you've started to eat. Whichever method works best for you is the method that you should choose.

A few details that you should record in your small journal is the amount of meals you've eaten per day, the size of each meal for every meal you've eaten for the day, the time of each meal, and your thoughts and feelings at every meal.

Basically, an easy way or organize those points in order would be time, size, thoughts or feelings, and amount. The reason why amount is last is because the amount is the overall of the day while the rest of the list is the individual meals of that particular day.

One way to set up your list would be making a small box. If you've ever used Microsoft Excel then you would know what I'm talking about.

Boxes and columns are your friends when you try to organize data. However, the method is entirely up to you.

Most people would prefer to keep a digital data of their progress. That is fine and when that normally happens, they would simply use their journal to jolt down notes of whatever information they wanted to record. By the end of the day, those notes would be typed out and sorted on the computer.

In the end, the method is really up to your personal taste. There are those who tend to record everything on their smart phones and there are those who prefer writing their data out on paper, or writing them on paper and transferring the data to their computers.

You have to think about what type of situation that you're in and how your life plays out.

Obviously, you are not going to pull out a phone during work even if you're allowed to eat. It's cases like these that will make you write your data down rather than typing them to a phone.

Overall, when you pick a method for yourself, pick one that you are comfortable doing and one that is convenient for you.

# Chapter 2 - Diet Facts

Here are some fun facts that you should know before running head on into the program.

Society has always lived on mainly by the word of mouth, which is mainly a "you hear it, you believe it." Newsflash, that's not a good habit to keep up.

There is some information that you can listen to and believe in and there is some information where you would have to do your own research.

This is one of them.

You've probably heard a lot about what to do during a diet and what to eat and what you should not eat.

You've probably already heard about the constant diet programs that are shown on TV.

You've probably already been through some of those programs or have done some type of dieting program that did now work for you.

A word of advice, if you don't follow a healthy program then your results will be much worse than what you've started with.

## Regaining Weight:

It is very possible to regain weight after going through your diet.

Whoever you've heard this from is correct. However, that shouldn't be the reason as to why you should give up.

In fact, the only reason why it is possible for you to regain the weight that you've lost is because you are not making any progress with the program.

You should already know that in order to lose weight you need to convert the fat in your body into muscle.

Therefore, if you are gaining weight, it means that you are doing something wrong with your diet plan and that you are converting your body muscle back into fat.

When you want to lose thigh fat, it's the same thing. Now that may sound slightly discouraging for you because no women want their legs to be full of muscle.

However, if you want to get rid of your thigh fat, you have to. It doesn't mean that you're going to end up with thunder thighs or something of the sort.

In order to achieve firm, thin legs, getting rid of the fat in your body is the best method.

Like the previous sections, it's not good to start being lazy after you've reached your goal.

It's very likely that most of you might start doing that, but it's highly recommend that you don't.

As I've said before, dieting is a lifelong program. It is a contract that you've signed on your own from the moment that you've started the program.

If you fail to continue on with the program like you have been doing then you will have to start from square one again.

Remember, it takes months to achieve the results that you want and it takes weeks to regain it.

What's worse is the fact that the second time around is even harder, which means that if you have to push your body to a second diet, it's going to take twice as much effort as before to lose the weight that you want.

Consistency will be your best friend in the diet program and so will dedication.

Don't ever let this fear of regaining weight drag you down. Fear is a negative emotion, which is something that you want to avoid.

It doesn't matter how physically healthy you may be and it doesn't matter how consistent you are with the program, if your mind is filled with negative thoughts then something will go wrong.

You will have to both be physically and mentally healthy. It is very possible to regain weight with negative thoughts so try to avoid it as much as you can.

**The Body You Want:**

As mentioned before, you will have to convert the fat in your body into muscle.

It is crucially important for you to mix and match your workout routine in order to maintain a balanced body structure.

If you want thin thighs, you will have to do more than one type of workout exercise.

It's very easy for anyone to hit the local gym and work on weight lifting. You need to, regardless, but it's not the only exercise that you can do.

In fact, it's preferred that you don't make strength training as your permanent workout routine.

If you do then you will only be gaining muscle. Your body will not be able to balance and, yes, you will get thunder thighs.

If you want thin thighs then you need to switch your exercise routines around. That doesn't mean that you try out a new routine every time you decide to exercise.

You want to be constant with what you are doing and at the same time, you want to change it up.

Consistency can only last for about 2-3 weeks when you're working your body. This is because 2-3 weeks is the average amount that your body takes to adjust to whatever you are doing.

We will get more into this topic at a later section but for now, you need to know that strength training exercises are not your only means of exercise.

There are different types of exercises that you need to practice in order to achieve the shape that you want.

Strength training exercises are weight lifting. When you lift weights, it's fairly easy for your body to gain muscles over a shorter period of time.

However, that is all you will be getting. Your body will start to bulk up and your muscles will build to the point where you can see it.

If you were aiming to be a body builder then it's fine, but that is obviously not your goal right now.

You want to achieve firm, thin thighs. In order to do that you need to work on both strength training and aerobics exercises.

Aerobics workout help improve your flexibility. It is the type of exercise that can help shape your body into the form that you want it to.

It is best if you were to combine the two types of exercises together when you work out.

Keep in mind that you would have to adjust the workout routine that you do every 2-3 weeks.

Lifting the same weights and doing the same aerobics exercises aren't going to cut it for you.

Also, once your body is used to exercising, rise up the intensity of the workout for better results.

Lastly, be sure to add some cardiovascular exercises. These are the types of exercises that improve your heart and lungs.

It's rather important for you to mix these exercises up with the exercises that you need to do.

It will help you greatly for more intensive workout.

Cardiovascular exercises depend more on eating healthy than the other types of exercises because it deals more with your heart and lungs rather than getting rid of your fat.

**Plateaus and Limits:**

Plateaus are a pain to stumble across by.

In life, you will come across many plateaus and you are expected to overcome with your own methods.

During this program, do not be amazed if you were to hit multiple plateaus along the way.

Since it is a lifelong program, be prepared to overcome all of the plateaus that you will have to face.

Most of the time, you will probably hit a plateau at least once every few months. Each time can be for the same reasons or it can be for different reasons.

The most common plateau that most people have trouble overcoming is when their body is no longer losing the weight that they want to lose.

Now that might sound as if they've reached their limit, but that's entirely different from hitting a plateau.

When you've hit the limit of the weight that your body can lose, you will know because your body will reflect on that.

When you hit a plateau, your body will also reflect on that and you will also know. There's no formula for figuring it out.

Anyone can simply look at you and figure out whether you've hit the limit or the plateau.

When you've hit your limit all you have to do is to maintain what you've achieved.

It's a lot easier than you think it might be because, by then, the daily routines that you have been doing will become a habit that you can't break away from.

By then your new comfort zone has already been established and by then, your cravings for unhealthy food will have settled down.

All you have to do in order to maintain your weight and figure is to keep doing what you have been doing.

Live your life as you have been when you were trying hard in the program.

If you want to change up some stuff then you are free to do so.

Just make sure that you never completely stop your diet program.

Breaks are acceptable but only up to a certain amount of time.

Plateaus are often harder to deal with simply because you have to start moving out of your comfort zone once again in order to make progress.

Usually, plateaus occur when your body has adapted to the routine that you are doing.

When that happens, it's necessary to adjust your routine into something new. It doesn't have to be the whole routine process just as long as you are making some changes overall.

It doesn't matter how well you eat or how much exercise you do, if your body has already adapted to the level of progress that you have currently then any results will be less effective.

There are two reasons as to how plateaus happen. One reason is the exercises that you are doing and the other is the food that you are eating.

This is why changing up routines are important because once your body has grown accustomed to your schedule, it will be hard for any improvements to happen.

When you exercise, try boosting up the intensity of your workout or try adjusting the workout that you're doing.

Often times, when the reason is your food intake, there are more details that you're expected to pay attention to.

You have to be careful as to what you are feeding to your body as well as how much you are eating.

Be sure that you are drinking water everyday, preferably up to 4-6 bottles a day.

Water is your friend. You might think that water may bloat up your body but what it's actually doing is trying to clean the inside of your body.

Water can improve your immune system and its zero calories to boot. So instead of busting out your usual juice or sodas, drink water. Tea is fine too but only if it's the natural ones.

**Overeating:**

It's very possible to overeat after a meal, which is why it's recommended that you eat slowly and not too quickly.

When you finish your food slowly you're also allowing it to digest within your body. You might feel full even before you've finished your food.

That doesn't mean you have to take half an hour to eat a small plate of food. You know that you're eating too fast when you can finish a plate of food in less than ten minutes.

Think about it. When you eat in a restaurant you wouldn't eat very fast now would you?

Take your time and eat at a slow pace. Your food isn't going to grow legs and run away from you, assuming that it's not alive that is.

Always eat breakfast. It's the most important meal of the day because it is the first.

You cannot expect that your meals will play out smoothly if you do not eat breakfast.

You also cannot expect your day to be completely normal like the rest because you decided that you wanted to skip breakfast for a day.

There are many reasons as to why you cannot skip breakfast. When you decide to skip your first meal of the day you are going to feel grumpy for the rest of the day.

You'll have a higher chance of having mood swings and you'll have an even higher chance of over eating on your next meal.

In order to stop yourself from overeating, it is best if you were to separate your meals into five different meal time a day.

You'll have three set meals - breakfast, lunch, and dinner - and you'll have two side meals, which will be between breakfast and lunch and lunch and dinner.

Your last meal should end with dinner. If you still feel hungry after eating dinner then wait for awhile after you've finished eating before eating an additional meal.

Be sure to make your last meal a light meal and be sure to eat dinner about three hours before bed. It will give your body time to digest the food rather than heading straight to bed immediately after eating.

Also, never treat yourself to a midnight snack. It can make you gain weight. If you feel hungry in the middle of the night then drink some water as a substitute.

It might give you a momentary feeling of fullness but it'll be enough until the morning.

With that being said, don't stay up all night either. If you aren't getting the proper sleep then your sleeping schedule isn't going to be the only thing that suffers.

# Chapter 3 - Exercising and Healthy Eating

In order to achieve thin thighs, you need to take control of your life and pay attention to the food that you're eating and the exercises that you're doing.

As mentioned before, you need to start planning a journal. That journal is going to contain records of your daily food intake and your exercise rates.

In addition, once you start your journal, you'll start to understand yourself a little bit more and your habits.

Most of the time, people don't realize half of the things that they do until someone has told them, which is why recording your thoughts and actions are important in being able to understand yourself.

Your journal doesn't necessarily have to be just a recollection of data that you have to record during your diet.

You can also write out your thoughts and feelings inside your journal.

There is no harm in doing that and since no one else is going to look at your journal besides you, your privacy will not be invaded.

In the beginning, you might not feel like recording anything more than your calorie intake and your exercise routines.

That is normal and most people would not go any farther than that.

However, it would be good to go the extra mile and jolt down some short notes about how you are feeling.

Either one is going to turn into a habit if you continue it long enough. Plus, it'll be good if you were to record your emotions along with your data.

It will be easier for you to notice your eating patterns and it'll be easier for you to find the issue of your eating habits in case if you were to reach a plateau and needed some answers.

**Healthy Eating:**

Eating healthy more important than exercise.

Yes, exercise is what allows your body to get rid of fat, but all of your health and successes are made within the kitchen.

Food is important for any type of diet. If you want firm, thin thighs, you're going to need to work harder than taking a simple trip to the gym.

You're going to need to eat healthy and you're going to need to abandon all unhealthy food from your life.

That doesn't mean that you're going to become a full fledge vegetarian. No, that's taking it too far and it is only an option to do if you want to.

You are going to have cravings and you are allowed to fill up those cravings, but only at a certain point.

You are going to crave a lot during the program but you need to learn how to manage those cravings.

It's going to take a lot of willpower at first but after a while, it'll flow out naturally from you.

Eventually, you'll start to fear certain foods that you used to crave and you'll start to want certain foods that you've never liked before.

Give it time and a little bit of effort.

A few points to remember when eating healthy are that you should stay away from processed food.

Processed foods are foods that are mainly stored in cans and maybe even bags. Most or all junk foods are considered as processed foods.

If you can't tell which foods are processed or not then the nutrition labels are your best friends.

Every type of food has a nutrition label unless if it's the vegetables and fruits that you can find in the grocery stores.

When you scan the nutrition labels, you can see the types of ingredients that are used to make the food.

Processed foods have more than three ingredients in a nutrition label with half of those ingredients containing words that you've either never heard of before or cannot pronounce.

If you can't pronounce it then don't eat it because it's not good for you.

You want to eat foods that provide you with low calories like whole grain foods or vegetables and fruits.

Your body also needs protein so make sure that you include those in your meals.

Yes, it is possible to obtain protein for your body without the need of eating meat. Try not to consume too much protein in one meal. Each meal should have more vegetables, fruits, or whole grain than foods that contain protein.

As mentioned before, try to balance out your meals so you can have a total of five meals each day.

Three main meals and two side meals is a good number. It's best to eat every 3-4 hours in order to keep your metabolism going.

Don't push your body and wait until you feel hungry to eat because that will increase the chances of you overeating later on.

Note that eating less will not improve your chances of losing weight at a faster rate.

The faster you lose weight, the more weight you will gain later on and the harder it will be for you to lose those weights again.

You actually lose weight when you eat, assuming that you are eating the proper amount that your body can handle.

If you eat too little, your body will think that you are starving and it will convert your muscles into fat, causing your body to hold more weight.

When you eat too much, your body will store those extra calories as fat and give you more weight.

This is why it's crucially important for you to be able to keep track of what you are eating and how much you are eating in total per day.

Lastly, stay away from any self-proclaimed dieting food. Those are the types of foods that say diet on the name like diet coke, or diet yogurt, etc.

Any processed food that states diet on it simply means that is not healthy for you. If you are eating them because they are low in calories then stop eating them now.

They might be low in calories but they are high in sugar. Not to mention that they start making you crave other unhealthy foods that you shouldn't crave at all.

**Sleep:**

You need to sleep. Sleep is important for losing weight. It might not seem like it because you are simply laying there without doing anything but it is.

When you sleep, your body is resetting itself for the next day. If you do not sleep then you can easily gain weight.

It is also possible for you to disrupt your eating schedule if you don't sleep.

You'll start feeling tired for the rest of the day and you'll be having constant mood swings.

What's worse, if you don't sleep, it can affect your mental healthy. You'll be having negative thoughts that you shouldn't have and you'll start craving foods that you shouldn't crave.

It's best to have at least seven hours of sleep per day, preferably eight if possible. Your body needs it and you need it.

Lack of sleep can also result into your habit of having midnight snacks, which will make you gain weight even more.

When you stay up all night you are bound to crave, especially because you're going to be too lazy to cook a meal for yourself.

Sleeping late isn't going to cut it either. Even if you have the right amount of sleep that you need to function, sleeping at an inconsistent time everyday isn't going to help soften the situation up.

**Exercise:**

There are many different exercising routine out there for you to choose from. You want to mainly focus on exercises that will give you what you want.

However, you also want to focus on exercises that will also improve your health at the same time because you can't actually do one without the other.

Well you technically can but it's recommended that you don't. You want the best results that you can get for your body and for yourself.

It's especially important to focus on cardiovascular exercises. They are extremely useful exercises that can help stimulate your heart and lungs.

Cardio exercises are the type of exercises that you can easily do for the rest of your life. Even the elderly do these types of exercises to maintain their health despite their old age.

The sooner you start the better because the longer you keep at it, the healthier your body will be.

Cardiovascular exercises also helps improve your immune system and make you less vulnerable to diseases. You'll also have less of a chance of getting a stroke or a heart attack.

There are many different cardiovascular exercises that you can commit yourself to. The basic and popular ones are running and swimming.

Running is the easiest exercise that you can possibly do because anyone can do it. Unfortunately, you will become sweaty when you start running and your body will be soar for the first few weeks but that is only because you are still a beginner at it.

Cardiovascular also help burn the fat inside of your body. You want to be careful though. These types of exercises can buff up your thighs so you have to make sure that you balance them with a few flexibility exercises.

When you do cardiovascular exercises you don't necessarily have change what you are doing but how much you are doing.

If you chose running as your exercise then you would want to increase the amount of how much you run over time.

Let's say your starting point was half a mile. So after a month of so you would want to increase that half a mile to a complete mile.

Keep doing this until you know you've reached your maximum amount. If you don't like running alone then get a buddy to run with you.

There has to be at least one friend you have that cares about their health as much as you do. Make sure that you don't try sprinting right when you start your workout, if you ever do.

Always stretch before your workout so you don't have to go through the risk of pulling a muscle during the workout.

Give your body a slow ten minutes start before actually moving at your maximum pace. Just like how an engine needs time to go at the maximum speed that you want it to, you have to give your body time before you can immediately charge into your jog.

After you finish your exercise, don't immediately sit down and relax. Walk around for about five minutes so your body can cool down from the workout.

Do not eat or drink anything right after you've finished working out. If you're thirsty, wait until you've finished cooling yourself down.

Always stretch your body before any type of workout. There's a higher chance of you accidentally pulling a muscle if you don't.

Also, stretching helps relaxes your tensed body and prepares if for whatever you are doing. You don't even need to exercise in order to stretch.

You can stretch anywhere and anytime. For the best results, do your stretches early in the morning, a few minutes after you've woken up.

Stretch all of the muscles around your body, especially your back. Try not to lean your body when you stretch. It's a bad habit to get into.

Note that you will be sore after a while because you might not be used to it but it will improve. There are two types of pain when you're stretching: the good pain and the bad pain.

You'll be able to know which is which when you actually do it. The good pain will make your body feel good in a way after you've finished that part of stretching and the bad pain will hurt while you're stretching.

Try not to go the extra mile on your first time. You can risk pulling a muscle.

When you stretch your body, make sure that you are stretching both sides evenly. It won't do you any good if one side is stretched longer than the other.

Rather, it makes your body feel uneven when you do that. Be sure to hold each stretches for about fifteen seconds and count them evenly.

When you exercise, pick a place where it's quiet and less polluted. You're going to be required to breathe in and out as you are exercising so you do not want to be breathing in polluted air.

Cardiovascular exercises require you to breathe in clean air. You do not want to be caught running at a place where there is smoke everywhere because when you breathe in polluted air, your lungs can and will be damaged.

A quiet area to work out is also good because there are less people around. It's recommended that you do your exercises early in the morning when people are still barely waking up.

The air is fresher then because of the small amount of cars driving by. If you live near a park then it's easier for you because you won't have to commute your way there in order to work out.

Combine some strength training exercises to your workout routine. Strength training exercises are actually more convenient and easier to do compare to cardiovascular exercises.

You have to stretch anywhere anytime anyways so stretching exercises aren't particularly an issue.

Strength training exercises can be done in your home and doesn't necessary require any weight lifting like you think it would.

The usual push ups and sit ups are good for a light strength training exercise. However, there are a few more exercises that are made to give you the thighs that you want.

Fortunately, they do not require any heavy training nor do they require you to hit the gym. It would be good if you were to buy some dumbbells for extra performance but it's not essential.

The workouts listed are just an example of what you can do to get rid of your thigh fat.

Remember, you have to balance it out with both flexibility and cardiovascular exercises in order to achieve the maximum results.

You can do these exercises in your living room and they are short exercises that will only require about fifteen minutes of your time each morning.

As a beginner, you do not have to exercise every day. Rather, it's recommended that you don't on your first few weeks.

This is because you want your body to get use to the exercises that you are doing. Also, you will feel very sore after the first workout so you do not want to immediately start exercising again with that pain surrounding your body.

**Split Squat**

Split squats are quite simple and easy to do. This type of exercise works out your legs more than your upper body.

If you wish to work on your upper body at the same time, you can lift dumbbells as you're doing your squats.

If not, you can even use your dumbbells as additional weight. You do not have to resort to using dumbbells if you do not want to.

However, if you do, it's good to start with a basic five pound and move on from there. It is a very easy exercise to do and is not at all tiring, but you have to know that your thighs will be very sore after your first workout.

Basically, what you are doing in this workout is simply walking in the same place.

You do not have to work with your hands but if you are not holding dumbbells then it's recommended that you leave your hands on your waists rather than dangle them.

To start, move one of your feet forward and slowly lower your body until both of your legs are making a 90 degrees angle.

Do not let your knee rest the floor. Hold that position for up to five seconds and bring your body back up slowly.

Repeat the process with your opposite leg. Both legs are one count so try doing about fifteen on your first try. You will be tired near the tenth one depending on your current state.

**Runners Lunge:**

Runners lunge is quite similar to the split squat in terms of positioning. The difference between runners lunge and the split squat is the fact that runners lunge requires you to fully bend your knees down.

In runners lunge, your knees do not have to be at a 90 degrees angle and your legs may touch the floor.

However, for runners lunge, you are to stretch your leg back and learn forward with your other leg.

Regardless, you have to maintain a straight back and the pressure of this workout is more tiring than the split squat.

Since you are allowing your body to completely touch the floor, it requires more strength to push your body back up, especially when you are doing it repeatedly.

It is like having to sit down only to get back up after a few seconds. This is what this workout is about.

Note that you should hold each pose for about 15 seconds before switching. Do not go too fast and keep a slow and steady pace.

**Squats:**

Squats can be very tiring for beginners, especially if you haven't been working out for a long time.

It is guaranteed that you will be sore after this workout. Even if the pain does not come immediately, you will feel it the next day when you wake up.

This isn't the typical squats that you would do when you have nowhere to sit down and you're practically supporting your body weight through your toes.

This is the type of squats where you have to keep your feet flat on the ground as you try to support yourself. Basically, this workout is going to look as if you were sitting on a chair that doesn't exist.

For beginners, it's best if you were to do this near a wall. You will have to keep your back straight for this workout so start by leaning yourself against the wall.

Give enough room between the wall and your feet and slowly lower your body until your legs form a 90 degrees angle.

Keep your back straight and hold that pose for about thirty seconds if you can.

Also, try stretching your arms out while you are in that position. Take note on how long you can hold it and try to improve it each time you do the exercise.

**Floor Bridge:**

Floor bridges require you to lie down on your back so it's best if you were to do this workout on a carpet rug.

Do not do this exercise on your bed. You want your body to lean on top of a flat surface and not one that you can sink into.

Before starting, you want to get into position. Once your body is straightened on the floor, bend your legs up, leaving about a one or two inch gap between your butt and your feet.

Slowly lift your hips up and hold it for about two counts before releasing.

If this workout is hurting your body then stop and try it again. If the pain continues then try to stretch out your body before starting again.

If the pain is still there then I suggest you skip this workout to a later date. Make sure that you are tightening your body as you are lifting your hips up.

When you are used to the basics of this workout you should start moving your legs around.

Basically, you are in the same position as you were before. The only difference between the more difficult version and the lighter version is the fact that you have to move your leg.

In this version, as you are lifting your body up, you have to stretch one of your legs out. Make sure that your leg is completely straight in the air. Hold that position for two counts then release.

Repeat this process with the other leg. Preferably, you should do about ten sets of this as a starting point with the completion of both legs as one set.

# Conclusion

Start learning how to be comfortable with your body even before you start the program because once you finish, you'll love it even more.

Remember to sleep for up to at least seven to eight hours a day so your body can reset itself for the next day.

Always maintain your posture.

Once you achieve those thin, firm thighs that you've been fighting for, start walking with your head up and your back straight.

You'll be more confident with your body and your posture will improve along with that confidence.